Contents

The purpose of this guide is to map the recommendations of the *Rehabilitation following acquired brain injury: National clinical guidelines* (2003) published by the Royal College of Physicians and the British Society of Rehabilitation Medicine, and the quality requirements of the *National Service Framework for Long-term Conditions* (Department of Health 2005).

Foreword

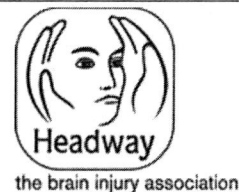

The effects of brain injury can be devastating. It can change everything in an instant, forcing people to rebuild their lives from scratch. Everyday tasks that most of us take for granted can suddenly become complex and challenging; entire futures can be lost and dreams shattered.

That's where Headway and associated professionals such as occupational therapists come in. It's our job to help people regain lost skills, adapt to their new range of abilities, while supporting them to achieve the highest level of functioning they can.

The value of occupational therapy in helping people affected by brain injury cannot be understated. It can play a pivotal role in helping people to rebuild their lives, giving them the tools and confidence to live as independently as possible. Indeed, many Headway groups and branches employ or work closely with occupational therapists as part of their personalised care and rehabilitation plans for service users.

A successful approach to helping adults with brain injury rebuild their lives should involve spending time with the client to learn and understand what makes them tick and what inspires them. It should mean establishing a set of goals for each individual client, taking into account their current abilities and future ambitions. Most of all, it should focus on what can be achieved – not what can't. Positivity should be at the heart of everything we do.

One of Headway's stated aims is to promote improved approaches to rehabilitation and community re-integration. To this end, we are delighted to support this guidance document. Anything that can help occupational therapists across the UK to provide a consistently high level of support to people with brain injury has to be welcomed.

Finally, a thank you to all occupational therapists working in the field of acquired brain injury. Working with adults with brain injury can be challenging and yet hugely rewarding. We know that there can be life after brain injury and we're grateful for all the hard work and dedication being shown by thousands of occupational therapists across the UK.

Peter McCabe
Chief Executive
Headway – the brain injury association

Acquired brain injury

A guide for occupational therapists

College of Occupational Therapists

College of Occupational Therapists

Specialist Section Neurological Practice

First published in 2013
By the College of Occupational Therapists Ltd
106-114 Borough High Street
London SE1 1LB
www.cot.org.uk

Author: College of Occupational Therapists
Editors: Donna Malley, Doreen Rowland
Project group: Jayne Brake, Anne Brannagan, Sue Bursnall, Gaynor Green, Verna Morris,
Ros Munday, Ruth Tyerman
Category: Guidance

British Library Cataloguing in Publication Data
A catalogue record for this book is available from the British Library

ISBN 978-1-905944-41-5

Typeset by Servis Filmsetting Ltd, Stockport, Cheshire
Digitally printed on demand in Great Britain by the Lavenham Press, Suffolk

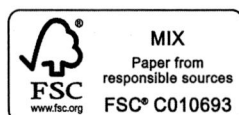

PART 1

Development and background to the guide

The purpose of this guide is to map the recommendations of the *Rehabilitation following acquired brain injury: National clinical guidelines* (2003) published by the Royal College of Physicians (RCP)/British Society of Rehabilitation Medicine (BSRM) and the quality requirements (Figure 1) of the *National Service Framework for Long-term Conditions* (Department of Health 2005). These are two of the key national documents which aim to improve the delivery of acquired brain injury rehabilitation services. It is essential that this publication is used alongside these two original source documents, which expand on the information and evidence base.

NSF for Long-term Conditions Care Pathway and the 11 Quality Requirements

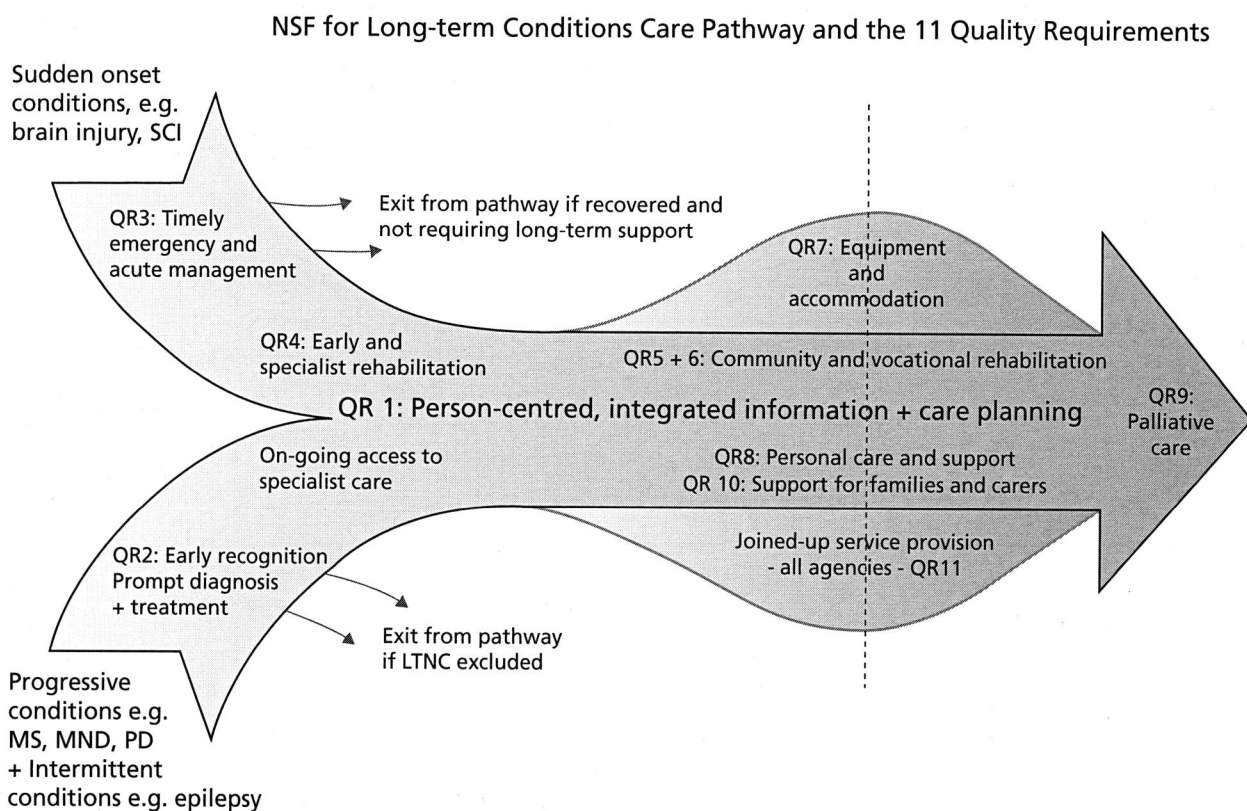

Figure 1: Revised version of the NSF for Long-term Conditions Care Pathway and the 11 Quality Requirements Fish Model (Adapted from Turner-Stokes & Whitworth 2005, *Clin Med* 5:3:203–6).

The publication has been developed as a practical guide for occupational therapists working with adults (over the age of 16 years) with a diagnosis of acquired brain injury. It is intended that the guide will enable occupational therapists to translate the published recommendations into clinical practice across the care pathway.

ii. Definition of acquired brain injury

The definition of acquired brain injury used throughout this document is that developed by the Royal College of Physicians (RCP)/British Society of Rehabilitation Medicine (BSRM).

Acquired brain injury is an inclusive category that embraces acute (rapid onset) brain injury of any cause, including:

* *trauma – due to head injury or post-surgical damage (e.g. following tumour removal)*

* *vascular accident (stroke or subarachnoid haemorrhage)*

* *cerebral anoxia*

* *other toxic or metabolic insult (e.g. hypoglycaemia)*

* *infection (e.g. meningitis, encephalitis) or other inflammation (e.g. vasculitis).*

(RCP/BSRM 2003, p7)

For the purposes of this document, stroke-specific evidence and guidance documents have not been included. It is, however, acknowledged that there may be significant overlap in the challenges facing people with acquired brain injury and stroke from an occupational perspective. Additional guidance regarding the occupational therapy management of stroke is available from the *National Clinical Guideline for Stroke: Occupational Therapy Concise Guide for Stroke* (Intercollegiate Stroke Working Party 2012).

iii. Overview of the role of the occupational therapist in acquired brain injury rehabilitation

What is occupational therapy?

Occupational therapy 'aims to enable and empower people to be competent and confident in their daily lives, and thereby to enhance wellbeing and minimise the effects of dysfunction or environmental barriers' (Duncan 2006, p6). Occupational therapists address such dysfunction 'using a range of interventions that often include adapting the demand of an everyday activity, altering the physical or social environment, teaching clients a new repertoire of skills or helping them to re-establish ones they have lost' (Duncan 2006, p7).

Occupational therapy is a complex intervention (Creek 2003) requiring the therapist to select an applied frame of reference, appropriate to the needs and goals of the client and the setting in which the intervention is conducted (Hagedorn 2000). Occupational therapists working within a rehabilitation setting use 'theoretical models as a basis for assessing, problem-solving and implementing a rehabilitation plan to enhance a person's occupational performance' (Doig et al 2008, p361). A core philosophy within the occupational therapy profession is that of client-centred practice and this should underpin occupational therapists' interactions with all clients.

What are the needs of people with acquired brain injury?

Non-progressive acquired brain injury can occur at any age, is usually of sudden onset, often has long-term consequences and impacts not only the person but their family and wider social and interpersonal relationships. Functional consequences of acquired brain injury involve complex interactions between biological, psychological and social factors, justifying a biopsychosocial model to guide assessment and rehabilitation. It is also necessary to recognise pre-injury factors (e.g. substance misuse, other medical conditions) and biological/physiological factors (such as endocrine dysfunction, sleep disorders, epilepsy) affecting function.

Following brain injury, a wide variety of physical and neuropsychological impairments can impact on activities and meaningful occupations while reducing a person's level of social participation, including their ability to participate in educational and vocational activities. These can include motor and sensory skills (including altered muscle tone, coordination, active movement, balance, proprioception, vision, smell and taste), communication (including language disorders and social communication), cognitive functions (including attention, memory, executive and metacognitive skills), emotion and behaviour regulation (including anxiety, depression, motivation, disinhibition and aggression). Additionally, mental and physical fatigue is commonly reported post injury. Neuropsychological deficits may not be obvious to an observer (a so-called 'hidden disability'), and people, therefore, commonly report feeling misunderstood and struggle to adjust to such deficits.

Contextual factors may also influence the practical consequences of acquired brain injury and the rehabilitation process; such as changes in roles, relationships and living situation. An individual's needs may be lifelong and can change over time, requiring reassessment. Occupational therapists are, therefore, well placed to work in partnership with the person and their family to help them to make sense of their injury and collaborate with them to develop and achieve personal goals through participation in a range of meaningful and purposeful activities.

Implications for practice

Multidisciplinary teams with expertise in brain injury are advocated by several documents that guide practice to meet the needs of service users and their families over the life course of their condition. Service user choice (including people with brain injury and their families/carers) and involvement in service delivery is a fundamental principle of these documents. There is a need for information about their condition and available services, in order to optimise autonomy and self management as far as possible.

Occupational therapy is delivered within a range of settings and is undertaken by professionals working alone, as part of a multidisciplinary team and with multiple agencies and services within the statutory, voluntary and independent sector. The overall goal of any rehabilitation process is to enable the person with the brain injury to increase their level of independence and social participation (including vocational rehabilitation), reduce their sense of isolation, support them to reconstruct their sense of identity and enhance their psychological wellbeing. Managing transitions between services can also present key challenges in multi-agency working.

As commissioning arrangements are changing, for example, within the NHS, there is a need to provide evidence that services deliver valued outcomes for people with complex problems as a consequence of acquired brain injury. While there is no one recommended outcome measure that adequately captures change in such a complex clinical population across the care pathway, Laver-Fawcett (2007) offers guidance regarding the principles of assessment and outcome measurement. The use of validated tools to support assessment and outcome measurement is particularly important to occupational therapy practice, where there is a lack of sufficiently robust evidence of the effectiveness of specific interventions within this clinical population.

iv. Aims of the guide and target audience

The aims of the guide are to:

• Support occupational therapists working with people with acquired brain injury in the implementation of the *Rehabilitation following acquired brain injury: National clinical guidelines* (RCP/BSRM 2003) and the *National Service Framework (NSF) for Long-term Conditions* (DH 2005).

• Guide clinical reasoning and clinical decision making while supporting safe and effective occupational therapy practice when working with people with acquired brain injury.

• Enable occupational therapists to critically review their own personal contribution and identify service and individual development needs.

The principal audience of this guide is occupational therapists working with people with acquired brain injury. It may also be of interest to people with brain injury, their family/carers, commissioners, other health and social care professionals.

v. Development process

This publication has been inspired by the Multiple Sclerosis Society and College of Occupational Therapists (2009) *Translating the NICE and NSF guidance into practice: a guide for occupational therapists.*

It has been developed by members of the College of Occupational Therapists' Specialist Section – Neurological Practice Brain Injury Forum in response to a request from their members for practical guidance.

Mapping exercise
Two main guidance documents relating to provision of acquired brain injury services in the UK were identified:

• The *National Service Framework (NSF) for Long-term Conditions* (DH 2005).

• *Rehabilitation following acquired brain injury: National clinical guidelines* (RCP/BSRM 2003).

Approval was received from Royal College of Physicians and British Society of Rehabilitation Medicine to create a guidance document for occupational therapists based on their guidelines.

The relevant sections for occupational therapy practice from the RCP/BSRM guidelines were identified and mapped against the quality requirements of the NSF Long-term conditions through consensus of the Brain Injury Forum Committee. This mapping exercise highlighted a need to establish an occupational therapy-specific evidence base in this topic area.

Identifying the key reflections for occupational therapists
Key reflective questions were developed to support clinical reasoning in each section of the document. These were based on the quality requirements, guideline recommendations and expert clinical opinion. The reflective questions were drafted and agreed by consensus of the Brain Injury Forum Committee and were subsequently ratified following peer review.

Consultation and peer review
Headway, the brain injury association, was consulted during the development of this guide, along with expert occupational therapy practitioners registered on the College of Occupational Therapists Specialist Section Neurological Practice database. Final approval was received from the College of Occupational Therapists' Practice Publications Group.

vi. How to use this guide

The information in each section of Part 2 of this publication is presented and ordered in the following way:

- The appropriate **quality requirements taken from the NSF** for Long-term Conditions.

- The **RCP/BSRM guideline statements** considered of most relevance to occupational therapy practice. (NB: The numbering in the RCP/BSRM section of each chapter correlates to that of the original guideline document and therefore may not always be sequential).

- The **key reflections for occupational therapists** to consider in terms of their own continuing professional development. These questions do not cover every eventuality but should encourage clinicians to think critically about their practice. This can be recorded in the checklist and action plan documentation provided in Appendix A.

- **Audit statements** to evaluate and evidence current practice are included at the end of each section. All the audit tools are also provided in Appendix B.

Each section has been written so it can be considered independently, enabling the reader to focus on one or more areas of practice at any given time.

This publication does not include statements from Section 9 (*The need for further research*) of the RcP/BSRM guidelines and Quality Requirement 9 (*Palliative care*) of the NSF for long-term Conditions as it was decided that these areas would be more appropriately covered by specific focused guidance into palliative care.

The following College of Occupational Therapists' documents should also be considered when reading this publication:

- *Code of Ethics and Professional Conduct* (COT 2010)

- *Professional Standards for Occupational Therapy Practice* (COT 2011).

The term 'person/people with acquired brain injury' has been used throughout this document except in those statements taken directly from the RCP/BSRM guidelines.

PART 2

Guidance, key reflections and audit statements

1 Principles and organisation of services

NSF for long-term conditions

Quality requirement 1: A person-centred service
People with long-term neurological conditions are offered integrated assessment and planning of their health and social care needs. They are to have the information they need to make informed decisions about their care and treatment and, where appropriate, to support them to manage their condition themselves.

Quality requirement 2: Early recognition, prompt diagnosis and treatment
People suspected of having a neurological condition are to have prompt access to specialist neurological expertise for an accurate diagnosis and treatment as close to home as possible.

(DH 2005)

RCP/BSRM Guideline

[This and all subsequent entries under the heading 'RCP/BSRM Guideline' are reproduced from: Royal College of Physicians, British Society of Rehabilitation Medicine. Rehabilitation following acquired brain injury: national clinical guidelines (Turner-Stokes L, ed). London: RCP, BSRM, 2003]

NB: The numbering in the RCP/BSRM section of each chapter correlates to that of the original guideline document and therefore may not always be sequential.

1. Principles and organisation of services

1.1 The provision of specialist services

G1: Every patient with acquired brain injury should have access to specialist neurological rehabilitation services:

- covering all phases from acute management, through medium-term rehabilitation to long-term support

- for as long as required – which may be life-long.

G2: Specialist neurological rehabilitation services for people with acquired brain injury should meet the standards as published by the BSRM and other professionals. In particular, they should comprise the following:

- a coordinated interdisciplinary team of all the relevant clinical disciplines

- staff with specialist expertise in the management of brain injury including a consultant specialist in rehabilitation medicine

- educational programmes for staff, patients and carers

- agreed protocols for common problems, such as management of spasticity, epilepsy, depression, etc.

1.2 Commissioning, planning and development of services

G6: Services should seek to ensure equitable access for all groups, and should be sensitive to ethnic, cultural, and religious issues.

1.3 Rehabilitation service networks

G8: Within the network of services, systems should be in place to ensure that:

- patients can be transferred between different services without any bureaucratic delays

- there is close communication and collaboration between local hospital, community and regional services to provide a seamless continuum of care

- patients with complex needs are able to regain access to specialised services as their needs dictate by referral through any appropriate agency.

1.4 Coordination of rehabilitation for individual cases within the network

G9: Within each service network, there should be a case management or equivalent system which gives brain-injured patients and their families/carers an identifiable guide and advocate through the whole care pathway.

G10: The individual or teams providing this 'case management' system should:

- register or be aware of patients with symptomatic acquired brain injury within their catchment area

- take responsibility for coordinating care and providing support and information for patients with acquired brain injury and their families from the time of injury, through the period of recovery and for as long as is required, to ensure continuity of care

- have knowledge of all the available resources for these patients and be able to advise patients, families, acute care providers, GPs and commissioners on the options available

- be able to access further appropriate professional advice and assessment as required.

1.5 Timing, intensity and duration of treatment

G11: Following acute acquired brain injury, patients should:

- be transferred as soon as possible to a rehabilitation programme of appropriate intensity to meet their needs

- receive as much therapy as they need, can be given and find tolerable

- be given as much opportunity as possible to practise skills outside formal therapy sessions.

G13: There should be recognition of the need for life-long contact to meet the changing clinical, social and psychological needs of patients and carers.

1.6 Staffing levels to meet demands for intensive treatment

G14: Staffing provision, in terms of numbers, qualification and experience in the management of brain injury, should be appropriate to meet the needs of the caseload.

G15: Within any rehabilitation setting, staffing levels should be sufficient to provide:

- safe lifting and handling of heavily dependent patients both for nursing care and in therapy sessions

- safe supervision for all patients, including one-to-one supervision where required

- adequate neuropsychological input to support the team in management of patients with cognitive and/or behavioural problems

- the full range of services offered by that unit

- a permanent staff establishment to ensure continuity of care

- a responsive service to support families in parallel to that for patients

- support and training for carers and rehabilitation professionals both within the service itself and in the community that it supports.

G16: Senior staff within each discipline should have specific experience in the management of acquired brain injury, and be of sufficient grade and experience to be able to guide and lead the rest of their team.

G18: Services providing community-based or vocational services function largely in the community and require a different staffing pattern with occupational and vocational therapists, as well as close ties with social, employment and education services.

Key reflections for occupational therapists

1. Do I work as part of a coordinated team to provide a person-centred service for people with acquired brain injury?

2. Do I have sufficient knowledge and skills to make reasonable professional judgements suitable to my level of responsibility?

3. Do I have the necessary skills/knowledge/competencies to meet the needs of people with acquired brain injury?

4. Do I offer an equitable service in terms of time, opportunities and resources?

5. Do I work to agreed protocols for common problems?

6. Do I base my practice on national guidelines and published evidence where possible?

7. Do I monitor the performance and quality of my practice and/or service against relevant local, national and professional standards and guidelines?

8. Do I use the results of my monitoring to improve my service?

9. Do I seek the views and opinions of people with acquired brain injury concerning their experience of the service I provide?

10. Do I work as effectively and efficiently as possible to be cost effective and to sustain resources?

College of Occupational Therapists
Acquired brain injury: a guide for occupational therapists
Audit tool

Date of audit		Auditor	Role
Location		Review due date	

1	Principles and organisation of services	What is your current practice? How do you evidence this?	Comments Action to be taken/by whom and when
1a	There is documentation about the provision of services for people with acquired brain injury, including: • specialist services; • commissioning information; • mechanisms for service planning and development; • rehabilitation service networks; and • coordination of rehabilitation for individual cases within the network.		
1b	There is documentation about the provision of occupational therapy services for people with acquired brain injury, including: • procedures for consent; • timing and intensity and duration of treatment; • staffing levels and competencies to meet service users' needs and demand for treatment; • equitable and timely access (and re-access) to services and opportunities for service user involvement in service design and evaluation.		

2 Approaches to rehabilitation

NSF for long-term conditions

Quality requirement 4: Early and specialist rehabilitation
People with long-term neurological conditions who would benefit from rehabilitation are to receive timely, ongoing, high-quality rehabilitation services in hospital or other specialist settings to meet their continuing and changing needs. When ready, they are to receive the help they need to return home for ongoing community rehabilitation and support.

Quality requirement 5: Community rehabilitation and support
People with long-term neurological conditions living at home are to have ongoing access to a comprehensive range of rehabilitation, advice and support to meet their continuing and changing needs, increase their independence and autonomy and help them to live as they wish.

Quality requirement 11: Caring for people with neurological conditions in hospital or other health and social care settings
People with long-term neurological conditions are to have their specific neurological needs met while receiving treatment or care for other reasons in any health or social care setting.

(DH 2005)

RCP/BSRM Guidelines

2. Approaches to rehabilitation

2.1 Teamwork and communication

G19: There should be a single interdisciplinary patient record system in which all members of the team record their interventions.

G20: A designated member of the team (e.g. a 'key-worker') should be responsible for overseeing and coordinating the patient's programme and acting as a point of communication between the team and the patient/family.

G21: All major decision-making meetings, e.g. assessment, goal planning, case conferences, discharge planning, should be undertaken by the relevant members of the interdisciplinary team, in conjunction with the patient and their family/carers as appropriate, and should be documented in the case records.

G22: Interdisciplinary protocols or integrated care pathways should be in place for management of common problems.

G23: Rehabilitation programmes should be developed in collaboration with family, carers or nursing staff to ensure that the programme is carried over into daily activities.

Acquired brain injury: a guide for occupational therapists

2.2 Goal planning

G24:   Goal setting should involve the patient and the family if appropriate.

G25:   Goals should:

- involve both long- and short-term objectives

- be meaningful to the patient and challenging but achievable

- be set at the level of whole team intervention as well as for the individual clinician.

G26:   Programmes and goals should be reviewed at agreed intervals and adjusted accordingly.

2.3 Assessment and measurement

G27:   All rehabilitation programmes should be monitored using tools which are appropriate, timely to apply and relevant to clinical decision-making.

G28:   Outcome monitoring should include analysis of goal attainment for each patient.

G29:   The team should have an agreed minimum dataset for documenting outcomes from the programme, and this should include:

- assessment tools which are shown to be valid and reliable

- reassessment at appropriate intervals

- regular audit and evaluation.

Key reflections for occupational therapists

11. Do I follow care pathways and protocols for assessment and management of common problems within my service?

12. Do I use appropriate assessments to identify individual needs?

13. Do I involve the person and family/carers in the goal setting process?

14. Do I provide information on the results of my assessment findings and plans for intervention to the person with acquired brain injury, family/carers and other members of the multidisciplinary team?

15. Do I develop the rehabilitation programme in collaboration with the person with acquired brain injury, families/carers and other team members?

16. Do I monitor and report evidence of occupational therapy intervention and outcomes? Does this include analysis of goal attainment, and impact on quality of life for people with acquired brain injury?

17. Do I use appropriate measures to evaluate both individual clinical outcomes and for service governance purposes?

College of Occupational Therapists
Acquired brain injury: a guide for occupational therapists
Audit tool

Date of audit		Auditor		Role	
Location				Review due date	

2	Approaches to rehabilitation	What is your current practice? How do you evidence this?	Comments Action to be taken/by whom and when
2a	There is written evidence of mechanisms in place to enable effective team working and communication between team members, the service user and their family and friends.		
2b	There is documentation to demonstrate client-centred goal planning, assessment and outcome measurement has occurred.		

3 Carers and families

NSF for long-term conditions

Quality requirement 10: Supporting family and carers
Carers of people with long-term neurological conditions are to have access to appropriate support and services that recognise their needs both in their role as carer and in their own right.

(DH 2005)

RCP/BSRM Guidelines

3. Carers and families

G30: Rehabilitation services should be alert to the likely strain on families/carers and, in particular, the needs of children in the family.

G31: Patients and their families/carers should be consulted with regard to treatment and care options and should be involved in planning of the patient's specific rehabilitation programme, negotiating appropriate goals, and in decisions regarding their care.

G32: Families of acquired brain injury patients should be offered timely:

- information and education about the nature of the brain injury, and about local and national services and support groups (e.g. Headway)

- referral to social services regarding their own needs

- assistance with the benefits system in relation to brain injury needs, including help to apply for appropriate benefits in relation to their own situation as well as that of the patient

- support and counselling to reduce distress and to prepare them for dealing with the attendant life changes. This support should be available long-term and be provided by professionals experienced in the management of brain injury and, where appropriate:

- the opportunity to learn skills, techniques and routines necessary to maintain rehabilitation gains

- information about the process of compensation for personal injury and approved sources of information concerning legal assistance, e.g. Headway Solicitor List and Association of Personal Injury Lawyers list.

Key reflections for occupational therapists

18. Do I establish the social situation of the person with acquired brain injury as part of my assessment?

19. Do I involve the family/carers in my rehabilitation planning to maximise independence and take account of their lifestyle and choices?

20. Do I offer information and education about the nature of the brain injury and its potential impact on the person's role, performance and function?

21. Do I consider the impact of the injury and its consequences on family/carers and provide them with necessary information?

22. Do I identify the family/carers' needs as part of the rehabilitation process? This should include how family/carers are coping practically and emotionally and, if required, help them to develop problem-solving strategies and/or signpost them to appropriate agencies.

23. Do I recognise the role of supporting agencies in order to offer current and relevant information to the family/carers?

24. Do I understand that different family/carers will make individual choices about their involvement in occupational therapy intervention?

College of Occupational Therapists
Acquired brain injury: a guide for occupational therapists
Audit tool

Date of audit		Auditor		Role
Location		Review due date		

3	Carers and families	What is your current practice? How do you evidence this?	Comments Action to be taken/by whom and when
3a	There is documented evidence that people with acquired brain injury and families/carers have been consulted and their views taken into consideration at all stages of the rehabilitation process.		
3b	There is evidence that opportunities for education, information and learning new skills are offered to families/carers in a timely manner.		

4 Early discharge and transition to rehabilitation services

NSF for long-term conditions

Quality requirement 2: Early recognition, prompt diagnosis and treatment
People suspected of having a neurological condition are to have prompt access to specialist neurological expertise for an accurate diagnosis and treatment as close to home as possible.

Quality requirement 3: Emergency and acute management
People needing hospital admission for a neurosurgical or neurological emergency are to be assessed and treated in a timely manner by teams with the appropriate neurological and resuscitation skills and facilities.

Quality requirement 4: Early and specialist rehabilitation
People with long-term neurological conditions who would benefit from rehabilitation are to receive timely, ongoing, high-quality rehabilitation services in hospital or other specialist settings to meet their continuing and changing needs. When ready, they are to receive the help they need to return home for ongoing community rehabilitation and support.

(DH 2005)

RCP/BSRM Guidelines

4. Early discharge and transition to rehabilitation services

4.1 Early discharge to the community

G33: Once a patient with acquired brain injury is conscious they should be assessed for all common impairments including:

- limb motor impairments, such as weakness, altered tone and incoordination

- bulbar problems affecting speech and swallowing

- sensory dysfunction which may impact on safety including:

  - hearing loss

  - visual problems, including reduced acuity, visual field loss, gaze palsies, etc.

- cognitive problems, especially impairments in memory, concentration and orientation

- language problems, especially aphasia

- reduced control over bowels and bladder

- emotional, psychological and neuro-behavioural problems.

Acquired brain injury: a guide for occupational therapists

G34: Any acquired brain injury patient being considered for hospital discharge should not be discharged until the following areas have been assessed by someone familiar with neurological disability, and all identified needs have been documented and met:

- presence of common neurological impairments, which should be documented

- safety in the patient's proposed discharge environment

- need for continuing immediate active rehabilitation and how this will be met

- risk to others – especially where children are involved

- awareness of the person and their family or carers of the current problems and how to manage them.

G35: Any acquired brain injury patient being considered for hospital discharge, or taking self-discharge, and who has not had an assessment by a member of the specialist neurological rehabilitation team, should be notified to that team and should have:

- preferably a fixed outpatient or domiciliary visit appointment with them

or, if this is impractical and problems are judged to be minor:

- a planned telephone contact from them within seven days.

G36: All patients being discharged after a recent acquired brain injury, regardless of follow-up arrangements already made, should:

- be given a card with details of the specialist neurological rehabilitation team and how to contact them

  - be warned of any likely problems they may face and how to manage them – including the fact that problems sometimes only become apparent some weeks or months later

  - have a family member or friend also informed of the above (with the patient's agreement).

G37: For all patients discharged after acquired brain injury from an acute hospital, the primary healthcare team (GP) should:

- be notified before or at the moment of discharge, with details of residual impairments and planned follow-up

- be given the details of the responsible neurological rehabilitation service to contact if problems emerge.

4.2 Transfer to rehabilitation

G39: Patients still in hospital at more than 48 hours with impaired consciousness or mobility should be reviewed as soon as possible after injury by a rehabilitation team to advise on appropriate referral and interim management techniques to prevent secondary complications such as pressure sores, contractures, malnutrition and aspiration.

G40: Severely brain injured patients still in coma should be referred to a specialist acute brain injury unit where their continued acute care may be supplemented by an interdisciplinary team of therapists trained in the prevention of potentially disabling sequelae.

G41: Those who are unable to go home directly and require a period of post-acute inpatient rehabilitation should be transferred to a specialist post-acute rehabilitation unit as soon as they are medically stable and fit to participate in rehabilitation.

G42: Patients transferring to rehabilitation services should be accompanied by their medical records or a full discharge summary including:

- a list of investigations undertaken and results

- details of any surgical procedures/interventions

- a summary of information given to the patient and their family regarding the nature of their brain injury and prognosis for recovery.

Key reflections for occupational therapists

25. Do I contribute to the assessment of level of consciousness?

26. Do I identify the impact of the person's abilities and impairments on their activities of daily living, overall occupational performance and safety?

27. Do I consider all factors associated with effective discharge planning and continuity of rehabilitation following referral to other services?

28. Do I explore relevant resources appropriate to the person's needs and intervention?

29. Do I identify any risks, including safeguarding vulnerable adults, ability to manage financial affairs and mental capacity, impacting on current intervention or future discharge planning and placement, and have I made appropriate referrals accordingly?

30. Do I provide a written report on transfer/discharge outlining assessment results, intervention received and outcomes and provided this information to relevant parties (with the person's consent)?

31. Do I provide the person with information on how to re-access/access services should their needs change over time?

32. Do I gain informed consent, before the person is referred to another service?

College of Occupational Therapists
Acquired brain injury: a guide for occupational therapists
Audit tool

Date of audit		Auditor	Role
Location		Review due date	

4	Early discharge and transition to rehabilitation services	What is your current practice? How do you evidence this?	Comments Action to be taken/by whom and when
4a	There is documentation to facilitate early discharge to the community and/or transfer to inpatient/specialist rehabilitation which includes: • results of assessments undertaken; • information about ongoing needs given to the person with acquired brain injury and their family/carers.		

5 Inpatient clinical care – preventing secondary complications in severe brain injury

---

NSF for long-term conditions

Quality requirement 3: Emergency and acute management
People needing hospital admission for a neurosurgical or neurological emergency are to be assessed and treated in a timely manner by teams with the appropriate neurological and resuscitation skills and facilities.

Quality requirement 4: Early and specialist rehabilitation
People with long-term neurological conditions who would benefit from rehabilitation are to receive timely, ongoing, high-quality rehabilitation services in hospital or other specialist settings to meet their continuing and changing needs. When ready, they are to receive the help they need to return home for ongoing community rehabilitation and support.

(DH 2005)

RCP/BSRM Guidelines

5. Inpatient clinical care – preventing secondary complications in severe brain injury

5.2 Management of swallowing impairment

G49: Patients presenting with features indicating dysphagia and/or risk of aspiration should be assessed by the interdisciplinary team for the most suitable posture and equipment to facilitate safe feeding.

5.4 Positioning and handling

G57: All team members handling patients should be taught safe and appropriate ways to handle patients.

G58: A suitable moving/handling programme for each patient with limited mobility should be:

- instituted through collaboration between physiotherapy and nursing staff within 48 hours of admission

- applied consistently by all staff

- reviewed and revised as the patient's needs change.

G59: Patients unable to protect their pressure areas should:

- have a clinical assessment for risk of pressure sores

- be provided with appropriate pressure-relieving equipment (mattress, cushion, etc.) without delay

- have regular inspections of the skin area at risk to ensure that adequate protection is occurring

- have access to specialist advice from specialist seating teams, tissue viability specialists, etc.

Management of spasticity and prevention of contractures

G60: Patients with spasticity should be assessed and treated by an interdisciplinary team with experience in the management of spasticity.

G61: Patients with marked spasticity and/or contractures should have a coordinated plan for interdisciplinary management.

Early sitting and standing

G63: Every brain-injured patient who remains unconscious or is unable to sit themselves up should have a graded programme to increase tolerance to sitting and standing.

G64: Patients should be stood and sat by adequately skilled staff with appropriately supportive equipment.

5.6 Establishing basic communication

G68: Assessment should include screening tests for hearing and vision, including the restoration of their usual aids such as glasses or hearing aids.

G69: Patients with severe communication disability, but reasonable cognition and language, should be assessed for and provided with appropriate alternative or augmentative communication aids.

G70: Staff should recognise that patients may communicate at a higher level with family and friends who know them well, than with professional staff.

5.7 Managing epileptic seizures

G73: Protocols should be in place for the management of acute seizures should they occur during rehabilitation.

5.8 Emerging from coma and post-traumatic amnesia

G75: Patients who demonstrate confused or agitated behaviour after acute acquired brain injury should:

- be assessed fully to establish the diagnosis and especially to rule out treatable causes including drug and alcohol withdrawal

- be managed in a quiet environment, avoiding over-stimulation

- have an agreed plan for behavioural management which is provided consistently by all staff.

5.9 Prolonged coma and vegetative states

G78: Where there is any doubt whatsoever about a patient's level of consciousness, assessment should be undertaken by a team with specialist experience in profound brain injury to establish the level of awareness and interaction.

G79: Where patients remain in persistent coma or minimally conscious states for more than three months, management in a specialist tertiary centre should be considered if the local services are unable to meet their needs for specialised nursing or rehabilitation.

Key reflections for occupational therapists

33. Do I understand the implications of avoidable secondary complications for people with acquired brain injury on occupational performance?

34. Do I have the knowledge and skills to contribute to the avoidance of secondary complications for people with acquired brain injury to optimise occupational performance?

35. Do I contribute, in collaboration with other health and social care professionals, to the assessment and management of:
    - safe feeding as part of the multidisciplinary team?
    - safe handling and positioning of people with acquired brain injury?
    - pressure care needs of people with acquired brain injury including specialist seating and cushions?
    - risk of developing contractures or abnormal posture as a result of spasticity, muscle shortening, joint stiffness, or reduced ligament length?
    - basic communication for people with acquired brain injury?

36. Do I have the necessary knowledge and skills to safely manage the person with acquired brain injury during an epileptic seizure?

37. Do I contribute to the assessment and management of level of consciousness and Post Traumatic Amnesia?

College of Occupational Therapists Acquired brain injury: a guide for occupational therapists Audit tool		
Date of audit	Auditor	Role
Location	Review due date	

5 Inpatient clinical care	What is your current practice? How do you evidence this?	Comments Action to be taken/by whom and when
5a There are occupational therapy protocols in place to facilitate preventing secondary complications for people with severe brain injury, which includes: • management of swallowing impairments; • positioning and handling; • management of spasticity and prevention of contractures; • establishing basic communication; • managing epileptic seizures; • emerging from coma and post traumatic amnesia; • management of prolonged coma and vegetative state.		
5b There is documentation to indicate that management of secondary complications has been considered and addressed and to identify any ongoing needs.		

6 Rehabilitation setting and transition phases

RCP/BSRM Guidelines

6. Rehabilitation setting and transition phases

6.1 Referral, assessment and review

G80: Each specialist rehabilitation service should have:

- a written procedure for referral and assessment to ensure appropriate and timely referral

- systems to deal with urgent referrals and to minimise waiting times for the service.

G81: The initial referral/assessment should routinely include:

- a full review of the patient's needs for rehabilitation and support

- an interview with the family/carers in order to:

  - establish their own needs

  - gain further insights into the needs of the individual within the home environment.

G82: The patient and family should receive:

- clear feedback of the results of the assessment and of the recommendations made

- continuing education/information about the nature and effects of brain injury.

G83: Following assessment, a written summary should be supplied to the referrer summarising the patient's rehabilitation needs with recommendations for further management.

6.2 Discharge planning

G84: Inpatient rehabilitation should continue while the patient requires the facilities, skills and therapeutic intensity of a specialist inpatient rehabilitation unit in order to make progress or while the hospital environment is needed in order to maintain safety.

G85: Patients may be transferred back to the community, once any appropriate specialist rehabilitation and support needed can be continued in that environment without delay.

G86: Planning for community transition should include:

• full preparation of the patient and the family

• assessment of the discharge destination environment and support available

• provision of any equipment and adaptations that are required

• training of carers/family in the use of equipment and in managing the patient to ensure patient safety in the home environment

• timely liaison with the community teams, primary care teams and social services to guarantee a smooth handover, agree an appropriate package of care and/or continuing rehabilitation programme

• graded discharge, usually with short-stay or weekend visits at home, to test the suitability of the home care arrangements

• giving patients and their families information about, and offering contact with, the appropriate voluntary services and self-help groups that may be useful to them, e.g. Headway, the Encephalitis Society, Different Strokes, etc.

G87: Transfer to the community should include a written care plan outlining:

• current needs

• key contacts

• responsible services/professionals

• sources of continued information, support and advice (e.g. Headway, Patient Advice and Liaison Service (PALS) and social services).

G88: Care plans should be agreed jointly between the patient and carer and health and social care professionals from the services involved in the transition. The care plan should be accepted by all parties prior to transition and a time-frame for review agreed – usually 3–6 months post discharge.

G89: Upon transfer or discharge, there should be a written report which includes:

• the results of all recent assessments

• a summary of progress made and/or reasons for case closure

• recommendations for future intervention.

G90: Copies of both the care plan and the discharge report should be provided to the patient/family where appropriate and all professionals relevant to the patient's current stage of rehabilitation, especially the GP.

Key reflections for occupational therapists

38. Do I know when I should decline a referral and how to manage this?

39. Do I identify family and carers needs or concerns as part of the assessment process?

40. Do I provide information on results of my assessment findings and plans for intervention to the person with acquired brain injury, their family/carers and members of the multidisciplinary team?

41. Do I know what to do when the person with acquired brain injury lacks capacity or ability to consent, e.g. due to low arousal, poor memory, communication deficits?

42. Do I provide the person with acquired brain injury and family/carers with information and education about the nature and effects of brain injury?

43. Do I provide appropriate training to family/carers to ensure they are competent in meeting the person's needs, including maximising independence and safety?

44. Do I know when a home assessment is required for a person with acquired brain injury?

45. Do I know how cognitive and behavioural problems may impact on use of equipment and adaptations in the home environment, and do I take this into account in my assessment?

46. Do I know where to source equipment to facilitate safe discharge?

47. Do I ensure that the person with acquired brain injury, family and carers are trained in the safe and effective use of any equipment and/or assistive technology I have prescribed?

48. Do I consider referral onto other agencies for funding for equipment and/or specialist assessment when appropriate?

49. Do I involve the person with acquired brain injury and their family/carers in identifying their needs on discharge from the service?

50. Do I support people with acquired brain injury and their family/carers to prepare for discharge from the service?

51. Do I know when to involve relevant agencies and services to facilitate a safe and smooth transition?

52. Do I provide information on appropriate voluntary services and self-help groups?

College of Occupational Therapists
Acquired brain injury: a guide for occupational therapists
Audit tool

Date of audit		Auditor	Role
Location		Review due date	

6	Rehabilitation setting and transition phases	What is your current practice? How do you evidence this?	Comments Action to be taken/by whom and when
6a	There are documented procedures within the service for: • obtaining and recording an occupational therapy referral; • declining and/or transferring a referral; • conducting an occupational therapy assessment; • review and mechanisms for discharge planning; • providing a written report on transfer/ discharge outlining assessment results, intervention received, progress to date and recommendations for future intervention.		
6b	There is evidence that these procedures have been instigated and the results documented and communicated in a timely manner to: • other team members; • the person with acquired brain injury; • family and carers with the necessary consent; • other relevant services on discharge.		

7 Rehabilitation interventions

> **NSF for long-term conditions**
>
> **Quality requirement 4: Early and specialist rehabilitation**
> People with long-term neurological conditions who would benefit from rehabilitation are to receive timely, ongoing, high-quality rehabilitation services in hospital or other specialist settings to meet their continuing and changing needs. When ready, they are to receive the help they need to return home for ongoing community rehabilitation and support.
>
> **Quality requirement 5: Community rehabilitation and support**
> People with long-term neurological conditions living at home are to have ongoing access to a comprehensive range of rehabilitation, advice and support to meet their continuing and changing needs, increase their independence and autonomy and help them to live as they wish.
>
> **Quality requirement 6: Vocational rehabilitation**
> People with long-term neurological conditions are to have access to appropriate vocational assessment, rehabilitation and ongoing support, to enable them to find, regain or remain in work and access other occupational and educational opportunities.
> (DH 2005)

RCP/BSRM Guidelines

7. Rehabilitation interventions

7.1 Promoting continence

Bladder management

G91: Patients who have continuing urinary continence problems should have:

- assessment by a professional trained in continence management in the context of acquired brain injury

- a regular monitoring programme

- access to specialist urologist/continence management and advice, including further investigation

- effective strategies for alerting carers to the patient's need to pass urine – in cases of communication and mobility problems

- an established toileting regimen based on reinforcement – in cases of cognitive impairment.

G95: Patients with continence problems should not be discharged until adequate arrangements for continence aids and services have been arranged at home and the carer has been adequately prepared.

Bowel management

G97:   Patients should be supported to sit up for defecation on a toilet or commode at the earliest safe opportunity, and at a regular time each day.

7.2 Motor function and control

G102:   The programme should include a written plan, with illustrations where appropriate, to guide other members of the team in carrying over motor skills into other daily activities.

Supportive seating and standing

G103:   Patients who are unable to maintain their own sitting balance should have:

- timely provision of an appropriate wheelchair and suitable supportive seating package

- regular review to ensure continued suitability of the seating system as their needs change.

G104:   Patients with complex postural needs should be referred to a specialist interdisciplinary team who have expertise in specialist seating.

G105:   Patients who are unable to stand independently should be provided with a suitable standing aid if appropriate, and this provision should be continued into the community if still required at the time of transfer.

7.3 Sensory disturbance

G109:   Patients with visual and/or hearing loss should be assessed and treated by an interdisciplinary team with the appropriate experience or in conjunction with another specialist service able to meet their special needs.

In the case of visual loss:

- opthalmologists should be involved in the assessment of vision

- orthoptists should be involved where there are problems with eye movement or double vision

- rehabilitation workers for the visually impaired should be involved regarding functional use of vision, mobility training and equipment.

In the case of hearing loss:

- audiologists should be involved in the assessment of hearing and suitability of hearing aids

- advice should be sought from a hearing therapist or social worker for deaf people, with regard to rehabilitation and equipment provision.

G110:   Patients presenting with persistent visual neglect or field defects should be offered specific re-training strategies.

Pain

G111: All patients should be assessed for pain on a regular basis and treated actively in accordance with their wishes.

G112: Staff should be alert to the possibility of pain in patients who have difficulty communicating and should pay particular attention to non-verbal signs of pain.

G113: Staff and carers should be educated about appropriate handling of:

- the paretic upper limb during transfers

- hypersensitivity and neurogenic pain.

G114: Protocols should be in place for management of pain which include:

- handling, support and pain relief appropriate to the individual needs of the patient

- review at regular intervals and adjustment in accordance with changing need.

7.5 Cognitive, emotional and behavioural management

Cognitive management

G120: Where cognitive impairment is causing management difficulties or limiting response to rehabilitation, specialist advice should be sought and, if appropriate, the patient referred to a formal cognitive rehabilitation programme.

G121: Patients with persistent cognitive deficits following acquired brain injury should be offered cognitive rehabilitation which may include:

- management in a structured and distraction-free environment and targeted programmes for those with executive difficulties (i.e. problems with planning, organisation, problem solving and divided attention)

- attempts to improve attention and information processing skills

- teaching compensatory techniques to overcome their everyday problems

- the use of external memory aids to enhance independence in the presence of memory deficits.

G122: Trial and error learning should be avoided in patients with memory impairment.

Mental capacity (competence)

G123: Patients should be assessed for their mental capacity to consent to procedures or to interventions which may carry significant risk or cause significant discomfort.

G125: Teams should consider the patient's ability to manage their own affairs, finances, etc. Appropriate advocacy/legal advice should be arranged for vulnerable patients to protect their best interests.

Emotional management

G126: Assessment of emotional state, including mood, should be undertaken in all patients, if necessary using specially adapted assessment tools.

G127: Patients should be given information, advice and the opportunity to talk about the impact of brain injury on their lives with someone experienced in managing the emotional impact of acquired brain injury.

G128: Patients should be provided with access to individual and/or group psychological interventions for their emotional difficulties, adapted to take into account individual neuropsychological deficits.

Behavioural management

G133: In the event of severe behavioural disturbance, appropriate supervision (including one-on-one supervision when required) by a professional trained in behavioural management should be provided to ensure the safety of the patient and those around him/her, and to provide effective behavioural management.

G134: Families should be given specific information and support to help them to understand the nature of cognitive and behavioural problems, and guidance on how to interact appropriately with the patient.

7.6 Optimising performance in daily living tasks

Activities of daily living

G141: All patients with difficulties in activities of daily living:

- should be assessed by an occupational therapist with expertise in brain injury;
- should have an individual treatment programme that is aimed at maximising independence in areas of self-maintenance, productivity and leisure.

G142: All daily living tasks should be practised in the most realistic and appropriate environment, with an opportunity to practise skills outside therapy sessions.

G143: Social services should recognise that provision of 'care' for some patients with acquired brain injury may mean the supervision and practice of community living skills, rather than hands-on physical care.

G144: Family and carers should be involved in establishing the most appropriate routines for activities of daily living which take account of their lifestyle and choices.

Provision of equipment/adaptations

G145: Every patient should be assessed to determine whether equipment or adaptations could increase their safety or independence.

G146: The need for equipment should be assessed on an individual basis and in the environment in which it will be used.

G147: Prescription of equipment should take account of any cognitive and behavioural deficits and their constraints on the patient's ability to use the equipment safely and appropriately. Where this is in doubt the equipment provider should be responsible for ensuring that arrangements are in place for regular review.

G148: Once an item of equipment has been identified as required for a patient:

- it should be provided as quickly as possible and *before* the patient is discharged to the community

- the patient, family and/or carers should be trained in its safe and effective use

- its ongoing use and relevance should be reviewed on a regular basis and in accordance with the manufacturer's guidelines

- patients should be given clear written information on who to contact for repairs, replacement, or for future help and advice regarding the equipment.

7.7 Leisure and recreation

G149: Community brain injury services should guide and support persons with significant brain injury in developing alternative leisure and social activities, in liaison with local voluntary organisations.

G150: All patients should be assessed by a rehabilitation professional or team to identify

- level of participation in leisure activities (including indoor and outdoor pursuits)

- barriers or compounding problems which inhibit their engagement in such activities.

G151: Patients with difficulty undertaking leisure activities of their choice should be offered a goal-directed community-based programme aimed at increasing participation in leisure and social activities.

7.8 Computers and assistive technology

G152: People with brain injury should be given information and advice about changes in technology and computer use relevant to their needs.

G153: Where necessary, a specialist assessment of each individual's ability to use a personal computer should be arranged and the need for adapted hard- and software recorded.

G154: Rehabilitation teams should:

- routinely consider the use of computers as an adaptive source of meaningful occupation for people with brain injury

- collaborate with other agencies (e.g. adult education schemes, employment schemes, charities, etc.) to obtain provision of adaptive hard- and software, and training to enable the individual to develop appropriate computer skills.

7.9 Driving

G155: The interdisciplinary rehabilitation team should:

- advise the patient and/or their advocate that they are obliged by law to inform the DVLA that the individual has suffered a neurological impairment and to provide the relevant information on its effects

- provide information about the law and driving after brain injury (e.g. the Headway booklet, *Driving after brain injury*)

- provide clear guidance for the GP and family, as well as the patient, about any concerns about driving, and reinforce the need for disclosure and assessment in the event that return to driving is sought late post-injury.

G157: If the patient's fitness to drive is unclear; a comprehensive assessment of capacity to drive should be undertaken at an approved driving assessment centre.

7.10 Vocational/educational rehabilitation

G158: Clinicians involved in brain injury rehabilitation should consider vocational needs and put patients in touch with the relevant agencies as part of their routine planning, and refer, where appropriate, to a specialist vocational rehabilitation programme.

G159: Patients seeking a return to employment, education or training should be assessed by a professional or team trained in vocational needs following brain injury. Assessment should include:

- evaluation of their individual vocational and/or educational needs

- identification of difficulties which are likely to limit the prospects for a successful return and appropriate intervention to minimise them

- direct liaison with employers (including occupational health services when available), or education providers to discuss needs and the appropriate action in advance of any return

- verbal and written advice about their return, including arrangements for review and follow-up.

G160: A patient requiring assistance in returning to previous employment should be discussed with the local disability employment advisor (DEA) with a view to a joint evaluation of vocational needs and/or referral on to a suitable vocational provider. When referring to the DEA, brain injury services should:

- provide summary information and explanation about the brain injury and its effects and about the rehabilitation input received to date

- attend the interview with the DEA to assist the patient in explaining about their work-related difficulties and to contribute to the development of an agreed joint plan of action.

G161: A patient who is considered to be capable of employment but unable to return to previous work or training should be referred, via the DEA, for employment assessment by a Jobcentre Plus work psychologist or other suitably trained professional experienced in assessment of vocational needs after brain injury.

G162: Patients considered to require a programme of vocational rehabilitation prior to work or training, should be referred either:

- to the DEA for assessment of suitability for referral under contract to a specialist brain injury work preparation provider, *or*

- direct to a brain injury vocational rehabilitation programme.

G163: In setting up a voluntary trial in the workplace, arrangements need to ensure the following:

- the requirements of the job match the skills of the patient

- the needs of the patient are communicated clearly to the employer

- health and safety training and insurance cover are provided by the employer

- there is appropriate support, including on-site job coaching when required

- the patient is guided and supported in adapting strategies to the workplace

- the trial is monitored closely through contact with patient and employer.

G164: In setting up placement into a long-term job, monitoring should be provided for at least six months to respond to any emergent difficulties, with follow-up thereafter to establish the long-term viability of the placement.

G165: Patients who are unable to return to employment or training should be provided with alternative occupational provision or adult education appropriate to their needs, as identified through joint assessment by NHS and social services or college of further education.

For more direct information on guidance related to returning people to work refer to:

- *Vocational assessment and rehabilitation after acquired brain injury* (RCP/BSRM 2004)

- *Vocational assessment and rehabilitation for people with long-term neurological conditions: recommendations for best practice* (BSRM 2010).

Key reflections for occupational therapists

53. Do I identify the impact of the person's abilities and impairments on their activities of daily living, overall occupational performance and safety?

54. Do I support the person with acquired brain injury to consider their needs in self-maintenance, productivity and leisure when developing rehabilitation goals?

55. Do I know how to deliver interventions and/or strategies to maximise the person's occupational performance?

56. Do I support the person with acquired brain injury to practise and develop skills within the most realistic and appropriate environment?

57. Do I support the person with acquired brain injury to practise skills beyond therapy sessions and into all aspects of daily living?

58. Do I establish the social situation of the person with acquired brain injury as part of my assessment?

59. Do I involve the family/carers when designing activities of daily living routines/lifestyle choices with the person?

60. Do I support family/carers and relevant others including MDT to use compensatory strategies in different situations?

61. Do I have the knowledge and skills to offer appropriate training to support workers to ensure they are competent in the delivery of rehabilitation programmes which maximise independence and safety?

62. Do I know how to seek and/or contribute to an assessment of the person's mental capacity?

63. Do I consider the impact of the person's performance deficits/impairments on their ability to manage their own affairs and finances?

64. Do I know how to accurately assess cognitive functions including:
    - level of orientation
    - arousal
    - attention
    - information processing
    - visual perception
    - memory
    - executive function
    - metacognition?

65. Do I know how to provide cognitive rehabilitation?

66. Do I know when to refer for more specialist cognitive rehabilitation?

67. Do I know how to contribute to assessment and management of mood and when to refer for more specialist intervention, e.g. psychological therapy?

68. Do I know how to manage severe behavioural disturbances and when to seek support for people with acquired brain injury and severe behavioural disturbance?

69. Do I know how to support family/carers to manage cognitive and behavioural problems?

70. Do I know how to seek support for people with acquired brain injury to talk about the impact of brain injury on their life?

71. Do I have the knowledge and skills to offer retraining strategies to a person with visual neglect or visual field deficit?

72. Do I understand how pain following acquired brain injury can impact on occupational performance and offer advice regarding pain management?

73. Do I assess the person's seating requirements, including provision of an appropriate wheelchair and suitable supported seating package?

74. Do I make referrals on to appropriate agencies according to my assessment findings, e.g. specialist seating services?

75. Do I ensure the person has appropriate and timely wheelchair assessment and seating provision with regular review?

76. Do I know how assistive technology and/or computer use may enhance the person's independence and quality of life and how to make appropriate referrals accordingly?

77. Do I ensure the person has an understanding of the process for returning to driving and any factors that might contribute to decision making based upon my assessment?

78. Do I know about services available for people with acquired brain injury regarding driving assessment and how to access them?

79. Do I consider return to work, training or study routinely as part of the rehabilitation process?

80. Do I know how to assess vocational and educational needs, including work history, job role, and the impact of impairments on return to work/education?

81. Do I support the person with acquired brain injury to develop an individualised return to work/education programme, including, where appropriate, on-site assessment, graded return and liaison with relevant agencies?

82. Do I know the relevant agencies and professionals involved in the return to work/training/education process and support the person with acquired brain injury to access them?

83. Do I know how to seek ongoing support for the person with acquired brain injury following their return to work?

84. Do I know how to support people with acquired brain injury who are unable to return to work or study to develop structure within their occupational lives?

College of Occupational Therapists
Acquired brain injury: a guide for occupational therapists
Audit tool

Date of audit	Auditor	Role
Location	Review due date	

7	Rehabilitation interventions	What is your current practice? How do you evidence this?	Comments Action to be taken/by whom and when
7a	There are documented, evidence-based occupational therapy assessment and rehabilitation protocols to promote: • continence; • motor function and control; • sensory disturbance; • cognition; • emotion and behaviour.		
7b	There is evidence of how occupational therapists within the service approach rehabilitation interventions to optimise performance of individuals with acquired brain injury in the domains of: • daily living tasks; • leisure and recreation; • computers and assistive technology; • driving; • occupational goals and vocational needs.		
7c	There is documentation to demonstrate that rehabilitation needs in these domains were identified and addressed, the outcome of interventions and ongoing needs of discharge from the service.		

Date of audit		Auditor		Role
Location		Review due date		

7	Rehabilitation interventions (continued)	What is your current practice? How do you evidence this?	Comments Action to be taken/by whom and when
7d	There is evidence that the occupational therapist has considered and provided information to relevant people about the person's cognitive function and behaviour and its impact on functioning in different domains.		
7e	There is evidence of an individual therapy programme which maximises independence and quality of life using recommended interventions.		
7f	There is evidence that the person has been provided with clear written information on who to contact for repair/replacement of equipment and/or assistive technology which has been prescribed.		

College of Occupational Therapists
Acquired brain injury: a guide for occupational therapists
Audit tool

Date of audit		Auditor		Role	
Location			Review due date		

7	Rehabilitation interventions (continued)	What is your current practice? How do you evidence this?	Comments Action to be taken/by whom and when
7g	There is evidence of referral to appropriate services to meet ongoing needs.		
7h	There is evidence of a comprehensive report outlining assessment results, intervention, outcomes and needs on discharge.		
7i	There is evidence of timely liaison with all the relevant agencies to facilitate a safe and smooth transition.		

8 Continuing care and support

RCP/BSRM Guidelines

8. Continuing care and support

8.1 General principles

G166: Patients with significant acquired brain injury should have long-term access to an individual or team with experience in management of acquired brain injury that:

- takes responsibility for their continuing care and support needs

- has knowledge of the various specialist and local services available

- co-ordinates appropriate referrals, assessments and reviews as required

- works across the range of statutory, voluntary and independent services to meet the needs of patients and their families.

G167: Care services should be provided by skilled workers, trained in the needs of acquired brain injury patients, to ensure that:

- the support is relevant and appropriate to meet needs

- care provision takes into account the needs of those with cognitive and communication problems.

G168: Family and carers should be:

- involved in assessment and subsequent decisions about help that is required

- offered assessment to establish their own needs and to increase the sustainability of the caring role.

8.2 Joint health and social services provision

G170: Community health and social services managers should work in partnership to ensure that an adequate range of services exists to meet the specific needs of those with acquired brain injury and their carers.

These should include:

- assistance with provision for respite care

- supported living arrangements, care home facilities, day centres, etc.

- equipment provision and maintenance

- assistance with claiming the relevant benefits for both patients and their families/carers

- access to continued healthcare and rehabilitation through regular review or through open access by self-referral

- brain injury education for families including information written specifically for children and siblings

- guidance and support for families in managing specific brain injury difficulties

- sexual and relationship counselling

- peer group support

- opportunities for purposeful activities including leisure and voluntary work.

G171: There should be explicit pathways for collaborative working between the various statutory and voluntary services including:

- primary care trusts

- social services

- housing departments

- education authorities

- employment authorities (e.g. Jobcentre Plus)

- benefits agencies

- advocacy services

- voluntary agencies

- driving assessment centres

- probation and the criminal justice system.

Key reflections for occupational therapists

85. Do I share knowledge and skills with those supporting the ongoing needs of the person with acquired brain injury?

86. Do I consider the need to access other agencies now and in the future and provide adequate information to enable the person to engage and re-access agencies as necessary?

87. Do I consider the holistic needs and requirements of the family/carers in relation to education support and guidance in all aspects of care and management?

College of Occupational Therapists
Acquired brain injury: a guide for occupational therapists
Audit tool

Date of audit			Auditor		Role	
Location			Review due date			

8	Continuing care and support	What is your current practice? How do you evidence this?	Comments Action to be taken/by whom and when
8a	There is evidence that the occupational therapist has ensured the person with acquired brain injury and their families/carers have information to facilitate timely referral/access to services available in the statutory, voluntary and independent sectors.		
8b	There is evidence that the occupational therapist has offered/provided training/ information to families and carers about brain injury to facilitate the care of the person with acquired brain injury.		
8c	There is evidence of partnership working across agencies as/when appropriate.		

Appendix A: Key reflections – checklist and action plan

1. Principles and organisation of services	Yes	No	Action / comment
1. Do I work as part of a coordinated team to provide a person-centred service for people with acquired brain injury?			
2. Do I have sufficient knowledge and skills to make reasonable professional judgements suitable to my level of responsibility?			
3. Do I have the necessary skills/knowledge/competencies to meet the needs of people with acquired brain injury?			
4. Do I offer an equitable service in terms of time, opportunities and resources?			
5. Do I work to agreed protocols for common problems?			
6. Do I base my practice on national guidelines and published evidence where possible?			
7. Do I monitor the performance and quality of my practice and/or service against relevant local, national and professional standards and guidelines?			
8. Do I use the results of my monitoring to improve my service?			
9. Do I seek the views and opinions of people with acquired brain injury concerning their experience of the service I provide?			
10. Do I work as effectively and efficiently as possible to be cost effective and to sustain resources?			

2. Approaches to rehabilitation	Yes	No	Action / Comment
11. Do I follow care pathways and protocols for assessment and management of common problems within my service?			
12. Do I use appropriate assessments to identify individual needs?			
13. Do I involve the person and family/carers in the goal setting process?			
14. Do I provide information on the results of my assessment findings and plans for intervention to the person with acquired brain injury, family/carers and other members of the multidisciplinary team?			
15. Do I develop the rehabilitation programme in collaboration with the person with acquired brain injury, families/carers and other team members?			
16. Do I monitor and report evidence of occupational therapy intervention and outcomes? Does this include analysis of goal attainment, and impact on quality of life for people with acquired brain injury?			
17. Do I use appropriate measures to evaluate both individual clinical outcomes and for service governance purposes?			

3. Carers and families	Yes	No	Action / Comment
18. Do I establish the social situation of the person with acquired brain injury as part of my assessment?			
19. Do I involve the family/carers in my rehabilitation planning to maximise independence and take account of their lifestyle and choices?			
20. Do I offer information and education about the nature of the brain injury and its potential impact on the person's role, performance and function?			
21. Do I consider the impact of the injury and its consequences on family/carers and provide them with necessary information?			
22. Do I identify the family/carers' needs as part of the rehabilitation process? This should include how family/carers are coping practically and emotionally and, if required, help them to develop problem-solving strategies and/or signpost them to appropriate agencies.			
23. Do I recognise the role of supporting agencies in order to offer current and relevant information to the family/carers?			
24. Do I understand that different family/carers will make individual choices about their involvement in occupational therapy intervention?			

4. Early discharge and transition to rehabilitation services	Yes	No	Action / Comment
25. Do I contribute to the assessment of level of consciousness?			
26. Do I identify the impact of the person's abilities and impairments on their activities of daily living, overall occupational performance and safety?			
27. Do I consider all factors associated with effective discharge planning and continuity of rehabilitation following referral to other services?			
28. Do I explore relevant resources appropriate to the person's needs and intervention?			
29. Do I identify any risks, including safeguarding vulnerable adults, ability to manage financial affairs and mental capacity, impacting on current intervention or future discharge planning and placement, and have I made appropriate referrals accordingly?			
30. Do I provide a written report on transfer/discharge outlining assessment results, intervention received and outcomes and provided this information to relevant parties (with the person's consent)?			
31. Do I provide the person with information on how to re-access/access services should their needs change over time?			
32. Do I gain informed consent, before the person is referred to another service?			

5. Inpatient clinical care – preventing secondary complications in severe brain injury	Yes	No	Action / Comment
33. Do I understand the implications of avoidable secondary complications for people with acquired brain injury on occupational performance?			
34. Do I have the knowledge and skills to contribute to the avoidance of secondary complications for people with acquired brain injury to optimise occupational performance?			
35. Do I contribute, in collaboration with other health and social care professionals, to the assessment and management of: • safe feeding as part of the multidisciplinary team? • safe handling and positioning of people with acquired brain injury? • pressure care needs of people with acquired brain injury including specialist seating and cushions? • risk of developing contractures or abnormal posture as a result of spasticity, muscle shortening, joint stiffness, or reduced ligament length? • basic communication for people with acquired brain injury?			
36. Do I have the necessary knowledge and skills to safely manage the person with acquired brain injury during an epileptic seizure?			
37. Do I contribute to the assessment and management of level of consciousness and Post Traumatic Amnesia?			

6. Rehabilitation setting and transition phases	Yes	No	Action / Comment
38. Do I know when I should decline a referral and how to manage this?			
39. Do I identify family and carers needs or concerns as part of the assessment process?			
40. Do I provide information on results of my assessment findings and plans for intervention to the person with acquired brain injury, their family/carers and members of the multidisciplinary team?			
41. Do I know what to do when the person with acquired brain injury lacks capacity or ability to consent e.g. due to low arousal, poor memory, communication deficits?			
42. Do I provide the person with acquired brain injury and family/carers with information and education about the nature and effects of brain injury?			
43. Do I provide appropriate training to family/carers to ensure they are competent in meeting the person's needs, including maximising independence and safety?			
44. Do I know when a home assessment is required for a person with acquired brain injury?			

6. Rehabilitation setting and transition phases (continued)	Yes	No	Action / Comment
45. Do I know how cognitive and behavioural problems may impact on the use of equipment and adaptations in the home environment, and do I take this into account in my assessment?			
46. Do I know where to source equipment to facilitate safe discharge?			
47. Do I ensure that the person with acquired brain injury, family and carers are trained in the safe and effective use of any equipment and/or assistive technology I have prescribed?			
48. Do I consider referral onto other agencies for funding for equipment and/or specialist assessment when appropriate?			
49. Do I involve the person with acquired brain injury and their family/carers in identifying their needs on discharge from the service?			
50. Do I support people with acquired brain injury and their family/carers to prepare for discharge from the service?			
51. Do I know when to involve relevant agencies and services to facilitate a safe and smooth transition?			
52. Do I provide information on appropriate voluntary services and self-help groups?			

7. Rehabilitation interventions	Yes	No	Action / Comment
53. Do I identify the impact of the person's abilities and impairments on their activities of daily living, overall occupational performance and safety?			
54. Do I support the person with acquired brain injury to consider their needs in self-maintenance, productivity and leisure when developing rehabilitation goals?			
55. Do I know how to deliver interventions and/or strategies to maximise the person's occupational performance?			
56. Do I support the person with acquired brain injury to practise and develop skills within the most realistic and appropriate environment?			
57. Do I support the person with acquired brain injury to practise skills beyond therapy sessions and into all aspects of daily living?			
58. Do I establish the social situation of the person with acquired brain injury as part of my assessment?			
59. Do I involve the family/carers when designing activities of daily living routines/lifestyle choices with the person?			
60. Do I support family/carers and relevant others including the MDT to use compensatory strategies in different situations?			
61. Do I have the knowledge and skills to offer appropriate training to support workers to ensure they are competent in the delivery of rehabilitation programmes which maximise independence and safety?			
62. Do I know how to seek and/or contribute to an assessment of the person's mental capacity?			
63. Do I consider the impact of the person's performance deficits/impairments on their ability to manage their own affairs and finances?			

7. Rehabilitation interventions (continued)	Yes	No	Action / Comment

64. Do I know how to accurately assess cognitive functions including:
  – level of orientation
  – arousal
  – attention
  – information processing
  – visual perception
  – memory
  – executive function
  – metacognition?			

65. Do I know how to provide cognitive rehabilitation?			
66. Do I know when to refer for more specialist cognitive rehabilitation?			
67. Do I know how to contribute to assessment and management of mood and when to refer for more specialist intervention, e.g. psychological therapy?			
68. Do I know how to manage severe behavioural disturbances and when to seek support for people with acquired brain injury and severe behavioural disturbance?			
69. Do I know how to support family/carers to manage cognitive and behavioural problems?			
70. Do I know how to seek support for people with acquired brain injury to talk about the impact of brain injury on their life?			
71. Do I have the knowledge and skills to offer retraining strategies to a person with visual neglect or visual field deficit?			
72. Do I understand how pain following acquired brain injury can impact on occupational performance and offer advice regarding pain management?			

7. Rehabilitation interventions (continued)	Yes	No	Action / Comment
73. Do I assess the person's seating requirements, including provision of an appropriate wheelchair and suitable supported seating package?			
74. Do I make referrals on to appropriate agencies according to my assessment findings e.g. specialist seating services?			
75. Do I ensure the person has appropriate and timely wheelchair assessment and seating provision with regular review?			
76. Do I know how assistive technology and/or computer use may enhance the person's independence and quality of life, and how to make appropriate referrals accordingly?			
77. Do I ensure the person has an understanding of the process for returning to driving and any factors that might contribute to decision making based upon my assessment?			
78. Do I know about services available for people with acquired brain injury regarding driving assessment and how to access them?			
79. Do I consider return to work, training or study routinely as part of the rehabilitation process?			
80. Do I know how to assess vocational and educational needs including work history, job role, and the impact of impairments on return to work/education?			
81. Do I support the person with acquired brain injury to develop an individualised return to work/education programme, including, where appropriate, on-site assessment, graded return and liaison with relevant agencies?			
82. Do I know the relevant agencies and professionals involved in the return to work/ training/education process and support the person with acquired brain injury to access them?			

7. Rehabilitation interventions (continued)	Yes	No	Action / Comment
83. Do I know how to seek ongoing support for the person with acquired brain injury following their return to work?			
84. Do I know how to support people with acquired brain injury who are unable to return to work or study to develop structure within their occupational lives?			

8. Continuing care and support	Yes	No	Action / Comment
85. Do I share knowledge and skills with those supporting the ongoing needs of the person with acquired brain injury?			
86. Do I consider the need to access other agencies now and in the future and provide adequate information to enable the person to engage and re-access agencies as necessary?			
87. Do I consider the holistic needs and requirements of the family/carers in relation to education support and guidance in all aspects of care and management?			
Score / 87	Total %		

Appendix B: Audit tool

College of Occupational Therapists
Acquired brain injury: a guide for occupational therapists
Audit tool

Date of audit		Auditor		Role	
Location			Review due date		

1	Principles and organisation of services	What is your current practice? How do you evidence this?	Comments Action to be taken/by whom and when
1a	There is documentation about the provision of services for people with acquired brain injury, including: • specialist services; • commissioning information; • mechanisms for service planning and development; • rehabilitation service networks; and • coordination of rehabilitation for individual cases within the network.		
1b	There is documentation about the provision of occupational therapy services for people with acquired brain injury, including: • procedures for consent; • timing and intensity and duration of treatment; • staffing levels and competencies to meet service users' needs and demand for treatment; • equitable and timely access (and re-access) to services and opportunities for service user involvement in service design and evaluation.		

College of Occupational Therapists
Acquired brain injury: a guide for occupational therapists
Audit tool

Date of audit		Auditor		Role
Location		Review due date		

2	Approaches to rehabilitation	What is your current practice? How do you evidence this?	Comments Action to be taken/by whom and when
2a	There is written evidence of mechanisms in place to enable effective team working and communication between team members, the service user and their family and friends.		
2b	There is documentation to demonstrate client-centred goal planning, assessment and outcome measurement has occurred.		

College of Occupational Therapists
Acquired brain injury: a guide for occupational therapists
Audit tool

Date of audit		Auditor		Role
Location				Review due date

3	Carers and families	What is your current practice? How do you evidence this?	Comments Action to be taken/by whom and when
3a	There is documented evidence that people with acquired brain injury and families/carers have been consulted and their views taken into consideration at all stages of the rehabilitation process.		
3b	There is evidence that opportunities for education, information and learning new skills are offered to families/carers in a timely manner.		

College of Occupational Therapists
Acquired brain injury: a guide for occupational therapists
Audit tool

Date of audit		Auditor	Role
Location		Review due date	

4	Early discharge and transition to rehabilitation services	What is your current practice? How do you evidence this?	Comments Action to be taken/by whom and when
4a	There is documentation to facilitate early discharge to the community and/or transfer to inpatient/specialist rehabilitation which includes: • results of assessments undertaken; • information about ongoing needs given to the person with acquired brain injury and their family/carers.		

College of Occupational Therapists
Acquired brain injury: a guide for occupational therapists
Audit tool

Date of audit		Auditor	Role
Location		Review due date	

5	Inpatient clinical care	What is your current practice? How do you evidence this?	Comments Action to be taken/by whom and when
5a	There are occupational therapy protocols in place to facilitate preventing secondary complications for people with severe brain injury, which includes: • management of swallowing impairments; • positioning and handling; • management of spasticity and prevention of contractures; • establishing basic communication; • managing epileptic seizures; • emerging from coma and post traumatic amnesia; • management of prolonged coma and vegetative state.		
5b	There is documentation to indicate that management of secondary complications has been considered and addressed and to identify any ongoing needs.		

College of Occupational Therapists
Acquired brain injury: a guide for occupational therapists
Audit tool

Date of audit		Auditor	Role
Location		Review due date	

6	Rehabilitation setting and transition phases	What is your current practice? How do you evidence this?	Comments Action to be taken/by whom and when
6a	There are documented procedures within the service for: • obtaining and recording an occupational therapy referral; • declining and/or transferring a referral; • conducting an occupational therapy assessment; • review and mechanisms for discharge planning; • providing a written report on transfer/discharge outlining assessment results, intervention received, progress to date and recommendations for future intervention.		
6b	There is evidence that these procedures have been instigated and the results documented and communicated in a timely manner to: • other team members; • the person with acquired brain injury; • family and carers with the necessary consent; • other relevant services on discharge.		

College of Occupational Therapists
Acquired brain injury: a guide for occupational therapists
Audit tool

Date of audit		Auditor		Role	
Location				Review due date	

7	Rehabilitation interventions	What is your current practice? How do you evidence this?	Comments Action to be taken/by whom and when
7a	There are documented, evidence-based occupational therapy assessment and rehabilitation protocols to promote: • continence; • motor function and control; • sensory disturbance; • cognition; • emotion and behaviour.		
7b	There is evidence of how occupational therapists within the service approach rehabilitation interventions to optimise performance of individuals with acquired brain injury in the domains of: • daily living tasks; • leisure and recreation; • computers and assistive technology; • driving; • occupational goals and vocational needs.		
7c	There is documentation to demonstrate that rehabilitation needs in these domains were identified and addressed, the outcome of interventions and ongoing needs of discharge from the service.		

College of Occupational Therapists
Acquired brain injury: a guide for occupational therapists
Audit tool

Date of audit			Auditor		Role
Location			Review due date		

7	Rehabilitation interventions (continued)	What is your current practice? How do you evidence this?	Comments Action to be taken/by whom and when
7d	There is evidence that the occupational therapist has considered and provided information to relevant people about the person's cognitive function and behaviour and its impact on functioning in different domains.		
7e	There is evidence of an individual therapy programme which maximises independence and quality of life using recommended interventions.		
7f	There is evidence that the person has been provided with clear written information on who to contact for repair/replacement of equipment and/or assistive technology which has been prescribed.		

College of Occupational Therapists
Acquired brain injury: a guide for occupational therapists
Audit tool

Date of audit		Auditor		Role
Location		Review due date		

7	Rehabilitation interventions (continued)	What is your current practice? How do you evidence this?	Comments Action to be taken/by whom and when
7g	There is evidence of referral to appropriate services to meet ongoing needs.		
7h	There is evidence of a comprehensive report outlining assessment results, intervention, outcomes and needs on discharge.		
7i	There is evidence of timely liaison with all the relevant agencies to facilitate a safe and smooth transition.		

College of Occupational Therapists
Acquired brain injury: a guide for occupational therapists
Audit tool

Date of audit		Auditor	Role
Location		Review due date	

8	Continuing care and support	What is your current practice? How do you evidence this?	Comments Action to be taken/by whom and when
8a	There is evidence that the occupational therapist has ensured the person with acquired brain injury and their families/carers have information to facilitate timely referral/access to services available in the statutory, voluntary and independent sectors.		
8b	There is evidence that the occupational therapist has offered/provided training/ information to families and carers about brain injury to facilitate the care of the person with acquired brain injury.		
8c	There is evidence of partnership working across agencies as/when appropriate.		

Appendix C: Further resources

• Useful organisations and websites

Brain and Spine Foundation
http://www.brainandspine.org.uk/history-brain-and-spine-foundation
Accessed on 08.02.13.

Brain Tumour UK
http://www.braintumouruk.org.uk/ Accessed on 08.02.13.

British Association of Brain Injury Case Managers
http://www.babicm.org/ Accessed on 08.02.13.

British Association of Social Workers
http://www.basw.co.uk Accessed on 08.02.13.

British Psychology Society
http://www.bps.org.uk Accessed on 08.02.13.

British Society of Rehabilitation Medicine
http://www.bsrm.co.uk/ Accessed on 08.02.13.

The Center for Outcome Measurement in Brain Injury
http://www.tbims.org/combi/index.html Accessed on 08.02.13.

Chartered Society of Physiotherapy
http://www.csp.org.uk Accessed on 08.02.13.

College of Occupational Therapists
http://www.cot.org.uk Accessed on 08.02.13.

College of Occupational Therapists Specialist Section – Neurological Practice
http://www.cot.co.uk/cotss-neurological-practice/cot-ss-neurological-practice
Accessed on 08.02.13.

Connect (Aphasia charity)
http://www.ukconnect.org/ Accessed on 08.02.13.

Different Strokes – Support for Younger Stroke Survivors
http://www.differentstrokes.co.uk Accessed on 08.02.13.

Encephalitis Society
http://www.encephalitis.info/ Accessed on 08.02.13.

Epilepsy Action
http://www.epilepsy.org.uk Accessed on 08.02.13.

Headway – The Brain Injury Association
https://www.headway.org.uk/home.aspx Accessed on 08.02.13.

Job Accommodation Network
http://askjan.org/   Accessed on 08.02.13.

Meningitis UK
http://www.meningitisuk.org   Accessed on 08.02.13.

Royal College of Physicians
http://www.rcplondon.ac.uk   Accessed on 08.02.13.

Royal College of Speech and Language Therapists
http://www.rcslt.org   Accessed on 08.02.13.

Scottish Acquired Brain Injury Network
http://www.sabin.scot.nhs.uk/   Accessed on 08.02.13.

Speakability (Aphasia charity)
http://www.speakability.org.uk/   Accessed on 08.02.13.

Stroke Association
http://www.stroke.org.uk/index.html   Accessed on 08.02.13.

United Kingdom Acquired Brain Injury Forum
http://www.ukabif.org.uk/   Accessed on 08.02.13.

UK Rehabilitation Outcomes Collaborative
http://www.ukroc.org/ or http://www.csi.kcl.ac.uk/ukroc   Accessed on 08.02.13.

Vocational Rehabilitation Association
http://www.vra-uk.org/   Accessed on 08.02.13.

• For finding evidence in relation to brain injury and occupational therapy

The Cochrane Collaboration
Supports evidence-based healthcare and systematic reviews
http://www.cochrane.org   Accessed on 08.02.13.

NICE Evidence Services
Evidence in health and social care
https://www.evidence.nhs.uk/   Accessed on 10.04.13.

OTdirect is a specific site with links to useful resources including search engines for
literature searching
http://www.otdirect.co.uk/resmain.html   Accessed on 08.02.13.

OTseeker is a database with abstracts of systematic reviews and RCTs relevant to
occupational therapy.
http://www.otseeker.com/   Accessed on 08.02.13.

British Association of Occupational Therapists and College of Occupational Therapists
http://www.cot.co.uk/   Accessed on 08.02.13.

• Other useful publications and health legislation

British Society for Rehabilitation Medicine (2010) *Vocational assessment and rehabilitation for people with long-term neurological conditions: recommendations for best practice*. London: BSRM. Available: http://www.bsrm.co.uk/Publications/
VR4LTnCv45fl.pdf   Accessed on 08.02.13.

British Society for Rehabilitation Medicine (2009) *BSRM standards for rehabilitation services mapped onto the NSF for Long-Term Conditions*. London: BSRM. Available at: http://www.bsrm.co.uk/Publications/StandardsMapping-Final.pdf   Accessed on 08.02.13.

Intercollegiate Stroke Working Party (2012) *National clinical guidelines for stroke: occupational therapy concise guide for stroke*. 4th ed. London: Royal College of Physicians. Available at: http://bookshop.rcplondon.ac.uk/details.aspx?e=250
                                                Accessed on 05.12.12.

Neurological Commissioning Support (2010) *Halfway through – are we halfway there? A mid-term review of the NSF for long term conditions.* London: Neurological Commissioning Support. Available at: http://www.ncssupport.org.uk/wp-content/
uploads/2012/01/571.-NCS-Half-way-through-60-page-document-FINAL.pdf
                                                Accessed on 08.02.13.

Royal College of Physicians; British Society for Rehabilitation Medicine (2010) *Medical rehabilitation in 2011 and beyond: report of a joint working party of Royal College of Physicians and the British Society of Rehabilitation Medicine*. London: Royal College of Physicians. Available at: http://bookshop.rcplondon.ac.uk/contents/pub320-b2f017c5-
09ef-42fa-a306-6f30956b9186.pdf   Accessed on 08.02.13.

Scottish Intercollegiate Guidelines Network (2013) *Brain injury rehabilitation in adults: a national clinical guideline. (SIGN 130)*. Edinburg: SIGN. Available at: http://www.sign.
ac.uk/guidelines/fulltext/130/index.html   Accessed on 10.04.13

Appendix D: Contributors and acknowledgements

This document was written by members of the Committee of the Brain Injury Forum of the College of Occupational Therapists Specialist Section - Neurological Practice:

Editors

- Donna Malley - Occupational Therapy Clinical Specialist, Oliver Zangwill Centre. Practitioner Researcher NIHR CLAHRC for Cambridgeshire and Peterborough.

- Doreen Rowland - Neuro Services Manager, Defence Medical Rehabilitation Centre, Headley Court.

Members of the Committee of the Brain Injury Forum

- Jayne Brake – Occupational Therapy Manager, JS Parker Ltd, Case Management and Rehabilitation Services.

- Anne Brannagan OBE – Complex Trauma Manager, Defence Medical Rehabilitation Centre, Headley Court.

- Sue Bursnall – Manager Occupational Therapy Services, Cambridge University Hospitals NHS Foundation Trust.

- Gaynor Green – Consultant Occupational Therapist, Neuro Rehab Christchurch Group.

- Verna Morris – Independent Occupational Therapist, Counsellor and Associate Lecturer Sheffield Hallam University.

- Ros Munday MBE – Therapies Practice Educator and Principal Occupational Therapist, St Georges Healthcare NHS Trust.

- Ruth Tyerman – Programme Manager and Head Occupational Therapist, The Community Head Injury Service, Buckinghamshire Healthcare Trust.

The Committee wish to thank the following people and organisations for their support in the development of this document:

- Dr Jenny Preston, Consultant Occupational Therapist, Douglas Grant Rehabilitation Centre for peer reviewing the document and for her support and guidance to the Editors.

- Karen Beaulieu MSc – Advanced Occupational Therapy Award Leader, University of Northampton.

- Dr Angela Birleson – Principal Clinical, Integrated Occupational Therapy Service - Middlesbrough, Redcar and Cleveland, James Cook University Hospital, Middlesbrough.

- Tracy Newton – Lead Occupational Therapist and Therapies Manager, Neuropsychiatry Service, St Andrew's Healthcare.

- Julie Phillips – Outreach Occupational Therapy, Nottingham Traumatic Brain Injury Service.

- Louise Seawright – Senior Occupational Therapist, Graham Anderson House, Glasgow.

- The Royal College of Physicians for granting permission to reproduce the guidance statements from: Royal College of Physicians, British Society of Rehabilitation Medicine. *Rehabilitation following acquired brain injury: national clinical guidelines* (Turner-Stokes L, ed). London: RCP, BSRM, 2003. www.rcplondon.ac.uk. Copyright © 2003 Royal College of Physicians.

- The Department of Health for granting permission to use extracts from the National Service Framework for Long-term conditions (2005). Contains public sector information licensed under the Open Government Licence v1.0. http://www.nationalarchives.gov.uk/doc/open-government-licence/

- Multiple Sclerosis Society for permission to develop this guidance document within the format developed for their publication: Multiple Sclerosis Society & College of Occupational Therapists (2009) *Translating the NICE and NSF guidance into practice. A guide for occupational therapists*. Published by MS Society. Available http://www.mssociety.org.uk/professionals/

- Headway, the brain injury association, for reviewing this document and writing the Foreword. http://www.headway.org.uk/

- Professor Lynne Turner-Stokes and *Clinical Medicine* for granting permission to use the Fish model. Adapted from: Turner-Stokes L, Whitworth D. The National Service Framework for Long-Term Conditions: the challenges ahead. *Clinical Medicine* 2005;5:3:203–6.

Consultation for this guide

- Members of the College of Occupational Therapists Specialist Section – Neurological Practice.

- Members of the College of Occupational Therapists' Practice Publications Group.

References

British Society of Rehabilitation Medicine (2010) *Vocational assessment and rehabilitation for people with long-term neurological conditions: recommendations for best practice*. London: BSRM. Available at: http://www.bsrm.co.uk/Publications/Publications.htm   Accessed on 20.03.2013.

College of Occupational Therapists (2011) *Professional standards for occupational therapy practice*. London: COT. Available at: http://www.cot.co.uk/standards-ethics/professional-standards-occupational-therapy-practice   Accessed on 05.12.12.

College of Occupational Therapists (2010) *Code of ethics and professional conduct*. London: COT. Available at: http://www.cot.co.uk/standards-ethics/standards-ethics
Accessed on 05.12.12.

Creek J (2003) *Occupational therapy defined as a complex intervention*. London: COT.

Department of Health (2005) *National service framework for long-term conditions*. London: DH. Available at: http://webarchive.nationalarchives.gov.uk/20130107105354/http://www.dh.gov.uk/prod_consum_dh/groups/dh_digitalassets/@dh/@en/documents/digitalasset/dh_4105369.pdf   Accessed on 10.04.13

Doig E, Fleming J, Kuipers P (2008) Achieving optimal functional outcomes in community-based rehabilitation following acquired brain injury: a qualitative investigation of therapists' perspectives. *British Journal of Occupational Therapy, 71(9)*, 360–370.

Duncan EAS ed (2006) *Foundations for practice in occupational therapy*. 4th ed. Edinburgh: Elsevier Churchill Livingstone.

Hagedorn R (2000) *Tools for practice in occupational therapy: a structured approach to core skills and processes*. Edinburgh; Churchill Livingstone.

Intercollegiate Stroke Working Party (2012) *National clinical guideline for stroke: occupational therapy concise guide for stroke*. 4th ed. London: Royal College of Physicians. Available at: http://bookshop.rcplondon.ac.uk/details.aspx?e=250
Accessed on 05.12.12.

Laver Fawcett AJ (2007) *Principles of assessment and outcome measurement for occupational therapists and physiotherapists: theory, skills and application*. London: John Wiley and Sons Ltd.

Multiple Sclerosis Society and College of Occupational Therapists (2009) *Translating the NICE and NSF guidance into practice. A guide for occupational therapists*. London: MS Society. Available www.mssociety.org.uk/professionals and http://www.cot.co.uk/publication/books-z-listing/translating-nice-and-nsf-guidance-practice-guide-occupational-therapists   Accessed on 24.01.13.

Royal College of Physicians and British Society of Rehabilitation Medicine (Tyerman A, Meehan M eds) (2004) *Vocational assessment and rehabilitation after acquired brain injury*. London: RCP/BSRM.

Royal College of Physicians and British Society of Rehabilitation Medicine (Turner Stokes L ed) (2003) *Rehabilitation following acquired brain injury: national clinical guidelines.* London: RCP/ BSRM.

Turner-Stokes L, Whitworth D (2005) The national service framework for long-term conditions: the challenges ahead. *Clinical Medicine*, 5(3), 203–6.